The Preliminary Practice of

Altar Set-up &
Water Bowl Offerings

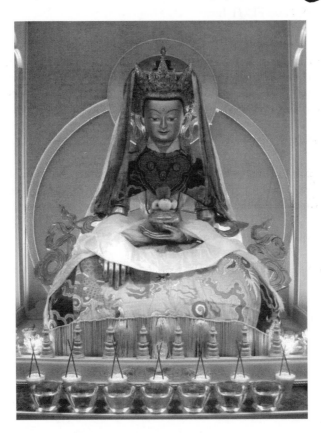

with instructions by Lama Zopa Rinpoche

FPMT Inc.
1632 SE 11th Avenue
Portland, OR 97214 USA
www.fpmt.org

ISBN-13: 978-0-9729028-4-7

Cover design by Lynn Shwadchuck. Cover photo of Shakyamuni Buddha in
sambhogakaya aspect in the gompa of FPMT International Office/Maitripa
College taken by Noah Gunnell. © FPMT Inc.

Set in Goudy Old Style 12./15 and BiblScrT.

Printed in the USA on 100% PCW recycled paper, FSC Certified.

Contents

Altar Set-up and Water Bowl Offerings

Walk into the meditation hall of any Tibetan Buddhist Dharma center or monastery and the eye is irresistibly drawn to the altar. Bursting with color and filled with stunning statues dressed in elaborate brocades, texts wrapped in traditional golden cloth, and offerings of saffron-colored water, incense, and flowers, the altar is designed to inspire the mind and move the heart. Most Tibetan Buddhist practitioners also keep altars in their homes, and a common question from beginning students is how to set one up for themselves.

Holy objects such as buddha statues, stupas, and texts are extremely beneficial to have. They inspire our practice and help us remember our goal of transforming our minds into compassion, peace, wisdom, and kindness. They also actually help purify our minds of negative emotions. When we see an image of the Buddha, a positive imprint is created in our minds. Later, that imprint or karmic seed causes us to be able to understand and practice the Buddha's teachings more clearly. When we practice well, our delusions and our suffering decrease, while our positive qualities increase. Eventually, we will eliminate all the negative problems and emotions in our minds and develop the positive ones to their highest potential; at that point, we become, just like the Buddha, fully enlightened.

In front of the images of buddhas and holy beings, we traditionally make offerings. The buddhas do not need these offerings, but from our side, this practice helps us learn to practice generosity. And by offering to the buddhas, we create a huge amount of positive potential (known in Tibetan Buddhism as merit), and this too nourishes our practice and study and helps us attain liberation from suffering and enlightenment as quickly as possible.

Creating Your Own Practice Space

It is very helpful for your practice to have a special room or space set aside in your home that is reserved just for practice. This is your "gompa" or "meditation place." The main items to go in your gompa are an altar, your meditation seat, and, perhaps, a text table and a bookshelf to hold your Dharma books. The altar is where you place the holy objects, pictures, and texts that inspire your mind. It should be used only as an altar and not double as a coffee table or desk, and it should be in a clean, respectful place. The objects should be placed higher than the level of your head as you sit facing your altar.

Before setting up your altar for the first time, clean the space well and burn incense to purify the place. After your altar and the rest of the space are complete, always keep the area clean. Sweep and dust every day before making offerings.

The Objects on the Altar

The Tibetan Buddhist altar contains a statue or photo of Buddha Shakyamuni and other deities with whom you feel connection. These symbolize the enlightened holy body. Photographs of your spiritual teachers may be included here as well. Traditionally, statues of the Buddha and other deities are placed at the center of the altar, with pictures of teachers placed to either side of the deities.

Statues of the Buddha and other deities need to be filled with certain mantras and incense and blessed. There are elaborate ways of doing this that require the aid of a tantric lama or someone well-versed in the process, and you will need this sort of help if you have a large statue, but there are also simple ways of doing it (see p. 37).

If you like, you may wrap each statue in a *kata* – the white silk scarf traditionally used for greeting and offering in the Tibetan Buddhist tradition. Wrap the scarf beautifully around the statue's base and part of the statue itself if you like.

If you have sacred paintings of deities (in Tibetan: *thangka*), these can be hung on the wall above the altar or on either side of it. Often, a kata is draped over the top of the thangka, or alternatively, wrapped around the decorative ends of the thangka at the bottom.

To the left of the Buddha as you face the altar, place a Dharma text. This symbolizes the enlightened holy speech. The text does not need to be written in Tibetan or Sanskrit; it can be a Dharma text in any language. Lama Zopa Rinpoche recommends placing the Sutra of Golden Light on the altar, and any other Dharma text may be used as well. Texts are often wrapped in yellow cloth or a brocade text cover before being placed on the altar. Cloth used to wrap texts should be new and clean, or at least never used for anything in the past except wrapping texts.

To the right of the Buddha as you face the altar, place a stupa. The stupa symbolizes the enlightened mind of the Buddha. The stupa doesn't have to be an expensive one –a simple clay stupa or even a photograph of one of the many amazing stupas from around the world are acceptable. If you have a real stupa, you might also like to wrap it in a kata.

If your altar is on one level, the order should be, from left to right (as you are facing the altar): text, Buddha, stupa.

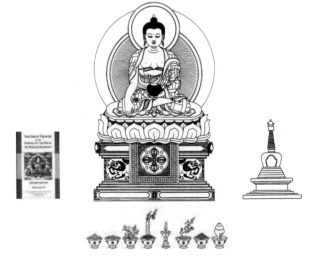

If your altar consists of three or more levels, the text should be placed highest on the altar, the Buddha statue on the next, and the stupa underneath that. Shakyamuni Buddha should be the central figure, and if you have other images, place them from uppermost on your altar to lower in the following order: root Gurus, yidams (highest yoga tantra deities, yoga tantra deities, performance tantra deities, then action tantra deities,) dakinis, and finally protector deities.

In addition to symbolizing the enlightened body, speech, and mind of the Buddha, the holy objects on the altar also symbolize the Three Jewels of Refuge. If you only have a statue of Buddha Shakyamuni, think that it symbolizes all Three Jewels. If there is also a scripture and a stupa, think that the stupa represents the Buddha, the scripture represents the Dharma, and the image of the Buddha represents the Sangha.

Offerings

In the Tibetan tradition, offerings are made on the altar every day. Offerings should be clean, new, and honestly obtained. Offer only fresh food and flowers, never anything spoiled or dirty. Fill bowls or vases high with offerings to create the cause for abundance; never offer a bowl that isn't filled to the top (for water bowls) or past the top (for food offerings). It is better to offer a small bowl heaped high with offerings rather than a large bowl that looks partly empty.

During the time of the Buddha, when someone important visited, they were offered them eight items as a sign of hospitality. In the 21st Century, we still offer very similar items to guests in our homes! These offerings are placed into seven or eight offering bowls at the front of the altar. From your left to right, they are: water for drinking, water for bathing the feet, flowers, incense, light, perfume, food, and music. Actual flowers, incense, candles or butter lamps, and food are offered in the bowls, while the rest of the offerings are represented with water. If there are only seven bowls, music is left off as a symbolic offering and is offered with the chanting of prayers and playing of musical instruments during prayers. If you are offering more than one set of offering bowls each day, as in the preliminary practice of water bowls, then all the bowls are filled with water – rather than filling some with the proper substances.

Setting Up Your Water Bowls

Traditional offering bowls may be obtained online and in many Tibetan shops. You may use these and may also use the many kinds of beautiful bowls available in the West, such as crystal dessert bowls or various glasses. Transparent colored bowls create an especially lovely effect. As long as the bowls are clean, you may use your creativity to its fullest in selecting bowls to use!

You will need containers for pouring the water into the bowls, a bucket or large container for collecting the water when emptying the bowls, and a towel for drying the bowls. All these should be used only for your water bowl offering practice and not for other purposes. Keep these items very clean and never place the towels or pouring container on the floor. Find a towel that does not leave lint on the inside of the bowls (if a brand new towel leaves lint, washing it a few times may alleviate the problem). Different towels may be more or less successful in drying the bowls, so you may need to experiment.

You will also need incense to purify the bowls and a safe place to keep the incense while it is burning. You may purchase a traditional incense holder from Tibetan shops, or may simply fill a glass with rice or sand and stand the burning stick of incense in that. If you opt for the glass and rice/sand version, be sure the ash will fall into the glass and not onto the floor, where it may burn carpet or wood floors or just create a mess!

Clean the room and then wash your hands before making offerings. Set your motivation that you are making these offerings on behalf of all sentient beings with the wish to attain enlightenment as quickly as possible to be of greatest benefit. Make three prostrations.

With a clean towel, wipe the bowls out three times clockwise (to dispel negativities created with body, speech and mind), and three times counter-clockwise (to bring to oneself the blessings of the Buddha's body, speech, and mind). Then pass each bowl over burning incense to purify it. As you fill each bowl with incense smoke, recite

OM AH HUM and think that you are filling all sentient beings' minds with enlightened wisdom, compassion, and power.

The most traditional way to offer water bowls is to begin with the newly incensed bowls stacked upside down to one side. Never place an empty vessel right side up on the altar as this represents offering nothing. With a pitcher of water, pour water into the first bowl until it is full. Then pour most (but not all) of the water from the first bowl into the second bowl and place the first bowl onto your altar, towards the left-hand side. Pour most of the water from the second bowl into the third, and place the second bowl onto the altar, just to the right of the first bowl. Continue in this way until all seven or eight bowls are on the altar in a straight line, each with some water in the bottom of it. This is called "seeding" the bowls. It is sometimes said that the pouring of the water from one bowl to the next in succession symbolizes carrying on the lineage of Buddhist teachings from teacher to disciple over generations.

If your bowls are too big to do the above practice or do not pour from one to the other without spilling, you may alternatively pour a little water into each bowl from the main pitcher before placing it on the altar. Regardless of which method you use, whenever pouring water into the bowls recite OM AH HUM. This is also true when lighting candles or incense to be offered. This recitation prevents disturbing spirits from polluting the offerings, causing obstacles to your practice.

Make sure the bowls have been placed in a straight line, close together but not touching. Traditionally, the distance between bowls is about the width of a grain of wheat. The symbolism in this is that if the bowls are too far apart, you may be creating the karma to be separated from your Guru. If they are too close together, there is the danger of complacency that comes with being too close to your Guru.

If possible, use saffron water in the bowls. Boil a pot of hot water and then put a small amount of saffron in the water. Cover the pot with a towel and let it sit until it is a deep orange or deep red color. Then place the water in a clean, covered container and refrigerate it. Each day, a small amount of this saffron water can be placed in the pitcher used to fill the bowls. The color of the saffron water in your bowls can vary – some teachers suggest it should be the color of a fine champagne, while others like the water to be a more vibrant yellow.

Now, use your pitcher of water and, while reciting OM AH HUM, fill each bowl. Pour the water like the shape of a wheat grain – in a thin stream at first, then gradually more, tapering off at the end. Try to pour the water without making noise and neatly, like a maiden of-fering tea to a king (as opposed to a barmaid pouring beer from the tap!). The water should fill the bowl to just about the size of a wheat grain from the top, so that the bowls are full, but not too full. If your bowls are not full enough, your wisdom will be incomplete; if they are over-full, your wisdom will be unstable.

In addition, you might want to cover your mouth with a kata or face mask as it is important not to breathe on the offerings as one is mak-ing them. Also, instead of water, one can offer flowers, incense, light and food in their respective places in the lineup of water bowls.

There is no limit to the quantity of either water bowls, flowers, lights, etc. that you can offer at the altar.

More Meditations for Water Bowl Practice

Lama Zopa Rinpoche has given various meditations to various people regarding what to think while doing the water bowl practice. These are not the only ways to do bowls, but are some options.

If your bowls are small enough that they may be held in one hand, the following meditation provides a way to accumulate merit and pu-rify negative karma all at once! Hold the bowl in your left hand and pour water into it with your right hand before placing it on the altar. The left hand represents wisdom and the right hand represents meth-od. Imagine that you are filling the bowl with oceans of nectar, and that your mind is filled with all good qualities, especially the specific qualities that you are currently trying to cultivate.

When emptying the bowls, the bowl held in your left hand repre-sents your mind, and the cloth held in the right hand represents the Dharma. As you pour the water out of the bowl, visualize that all your negativities – or a specific negativity that you are trying to eliminate – are completely removed from your mental continuum. As you dry the bowl, think that you are wiping your mind clean with the Dharma. As you incense the bowl, recite OM AH HUM three times and think that your mind is completely purified.

Similarly, one may do the above meditation thinking that one is purifying all sentient beings of their negativities and giving them all good qualities, or that sentient beings in each realm receive all they need for temporal and ultimate happiness. In the latter case, each bowl can represent one realm, with the seventh bowl representing the intermediate state.

While emptying and drying the bowls, you may recite the long or short Vajrasattva mantra to increase the purifying effect.

Presenting the Offerings

An Extensive Offering Practice (p. 25) can be used as a basis for performing your offering practice in an extensive way.

To perform your offerings in a simple way, generate bodhichitta, place your hands in the mudra of prostration, recite OM AH HUM three times, and imagine that your offerings are received by all the holy objects, statues, and scriptures in your gompa that are manifestations of the Guru's holy mind. Imagine that they experience great bliss. Then think that the offerings are received by the entire merit field, all the Buddha, Dharma, and Sangha, statues, stupas, and scriptures of the ten directions.

With the understanding that all these holy objects are manifestations of the Guru, imagine that the offerings are received and that the Guru's holy mind experiences great bliss. The three essential steps are: prostrating, offering, and generating great bliss in the holy mind.

After you have made your offerings, dedicate the merit for the swift enlightenment of all sentient beings.

Removing the Offerings

At the end of the day, empty the bowls one by one (from right to left) and stack them upside down or put them away. Never leave empty bowls right side up on the altar. Offerings should be discarded carefully

- water should be offered to plants or a garden or placed somewhere where it will not be stepped over. Flowers should be put in a clean place outside. Food may be left on the altar for a few days and then can be eaten or put in a clean place outside as well.

If you choose to eat the food that was offered on your altar, say the following mantra seven times to avoid accumulating the karma of stealing from the Triple Gem.

TADYATHA IDAM PENI RATNA PEMANI PARATNA NI SVAHA (7x)

Then blow on the food.

When to Fill and Empty Water Bowls

Traditionally, water bowls are filled as part of your morning practice and emptied in the late afternoon or early evening (before darkness falls). However, Lama Zopa Rinpoche does extensive offering practice every day, and he includes all the offerings set out in every center of his Dharma organization, the FPMT, and in the homes of his students. In addition, Rinpoche has invited students to also visualize these offerings as they do the extensive offering practice. Since Rinpoche does practices twenty-four hours a day, it is impossible to know when the extensive offering practice will be done. Therefore, in the many centers of FPMT, the bowls are set up twenty-four hours a day. This is the tradition of Lama Zopa Rinpoche.

Therefore, the bowls are emptied and immediately filled again in the mornings. However, if students choose to practice like this rather than the traditional way, it is important to think that these offerings are being offered by Rinpoche and others in their practice, and not just to do it like this because you can't bother to empty the bowls in the evening. In a center with the resident geshe who feels strongly that the bowls should be emptied before dark, the practice should definitely be done in the traditional way, according to the geshe's advice.

The Practice of Making Offerings

by Lama Zopa Rinpoche

Offering is specifically a remedy for miserliness. The result is to have control over sense enjoyments, as Lama Tsongkhapa had, so that sense enjoyments cannot disturb one. One will receive whatever one is seeking. During initiations, when offerings are made to the vajra disciple, particularly during the preparation, it is to be understood that from that time on any sense enjoyments can be utilized to develop bliss and voidness within oneself without them becoming a cause of suffering, without the mind being stained by samsara. That means without the sense enjoyments becoming the cause for craving to arise; rather, becoming the skillful means to generate bliss/voidness, and so to quickly cut off the dual view.

Similarly, when one makes offerings to the triple gem especially in maha-anuttara yoga tantra practice, they are made with the pure appearance of them having the nature of bliss and voidness. That becomes a method to quickly complete the two types of merit and become enlightened, after which all sense objects have a pure appearance, nothing appears as ugly or undesirable. Any form is beautiful, any sound interesting, any taste in the nature of great bliss. Anything that appears, appears in purity. Doing the offering practice in this way becomes the cause of achieving that result.

When performing offerings, you can offer to the merit field not only those offerings you have made at the altar and those mentally transformed, but also you can offer all the beautiful flowers, lakes, parks, the sun and moon – all the beautiful things, which are your own karmic appearance, the various sense objects you see in your view. You can think of all of those. When you offer light, you need not necessarily think of only the one or two butter-lamps you have lit, but however many lights you have on in your room. The clearer and brighter the light is, the better the offering. If it dispels more darkness the effect is greater. The external effect is greater so the inner effect of dispelling ignorance and developing wisdom is greater

When I travel, especially when I stay in hotels, I think it is a waste to not use all the lights! Especially if the place is cold it helps in keeping warm! Anyway, one has to pay for however many days one stays, so this is a way to make great business in accumulating inconceivable merit for much temporal and ultimate happiness! You can offer as many lights as you can see in the rooms.

Make offerings to every single holy object and every actual living bodhisattva and buddha in the ten directions. That also includes the many holy objects such as pictures and statues found in every practitioner's room. Firstly, making one offering to one buddha has unbelievable merit. And secondly, as I explained before, the internal phenomenon of karma is much more expandable in comparison to external things. I have given the example of how from one small bodhi tree seed thousands of branches and thousands of thousands of seeds come, but that is nothing compared to how karma expands. So each time you make an offering of even one tiny flower, or one incense stick, think that you are making an offering to every single holy object and actual living holy beings in all ten directions.

Offerings in Relation to Tantric Practice

When making offerings to the triple gem you can think like this: as you are generally performing the practice of offering in relation to tantra, specifically maha-anuttara yoga tantra, you yourself are the deity in the nature of the transcendental wisdom of non-dual bliss and voidness. The light or whatever you are offering is purified in shunyata, becomes emptiness, and becomes a pure offering having three qualities, which you may remember from the explanations on offering in maha-anuttara yoga tantra. I think the three qualities are similar in kriya tantra. Anyway, that can be understood from the prayer. You can think that the light, which is the transcendental wisdom of non-dual bliss and voidness, dispels all sentient beings' wrong conceptions and darkness of ignorance, and eliminates their two obscurations and generates the whole path in their minds. Similarly with incense: the incense becomes emptiness and then you see it as a pure offering – the incense of transcendental wisdom of non-dual bliss and voidness. Its scent purifies the sentient beings' two obscurations and generates the whole path and enlightens them in the essence of the deity that one is practicing. That is in relation to the sentient beings. Regarding the holy objects, it generates infinite bliss in their holy minds.

Water Bowl Offerings

His Holiness Serkong Tsenshab Rinpoche explained to us during the Jorchö commentary that when you clean the bowls you should use a clean towel. The significance of offering seven water bowls is to create the cause to achieve the seven limbs, or aspects, or qualities of the Vajradhara state – enlightenment. But that does not mean that you cannot offer more, that offering more is some kind of interference!

If you do not have many water bowls it does not matter. The ascetic meditators used their own wooden food bowl. I think it was Je Drukhangpa, a lineage lama of lam-rim, the guru of Phurchog Jamgön Rinpoche, and who is regarded as an embodiment of Maitreya Buddha, who lived an ascetic life practicing in a cave. He did not own texts and the necessary robes – the chögu and dingwa – nor did he keep many material possessions. When he ate, he took his bowl from the altar and ate his food from that. Then he cleaned it well and filled it with water and offered it at the altar. For those living ascetic lives, not keeping many possessions has a great purpose. If one is not living a strictly ascetic life, one should use one's possessions to accumulate as much merit as possible; then one is taking the essence from that which is essenceless.

When cleaning the bowls what you should think is the same as when cleaning the room. I do not remember word for word what Rinpoche explained. However, when one cleans the room, one should think that the broom represents method and wisdom, the whole path to enlightenment. So think the same in regard to the towel, and you can think that you are purifying the two obscurations of yourself as well as all sentient beings. If you have incense, light it and hold the bowls over it as a purification. Then stack the bowls.

Before putting the bowls on the altar you should put some water in them. There is a reason for this. You may have read Milarepa's life-story. When Milarepa made an offering to Marpa of, I think, a big copper pot, he offered it empty. It is said that he had to live on only nettles and bear great hardships in regard to food and the necessities of life because of the dependent arising due to that inauspicious offering. Marpa, knowing that it was a little inauspicious used a skillful method and asked Mila to fill the pot with butter and wax and make a light offering. That auspicious offering was the cause for Milarepa to be able to realize shunyata and generate the clear light and illusory body in that life. One can understand the purpose from stories like that; otherwise it looks like nothing more than just a rule saying one has to do this and this. So, you should not put empty containers in front of the altar; similarly, when you make offerings to the virtuous teachers put something in the container.

Fill one bowl with water, then pour most of it from that one into the next bowl, keeping a little in the first. Then again from the second one pour most into the third, keeping a little in the second. After you have put some water in the last bowl recite OM AH HUM three times to bless the water, the same as with the inner offering.

If you are a gelong (fully ordained monk) and offering incense, you should immediately remember: I'm doing this for Dharma practice; I'm doing it for other sentient beings. The reason for remembering at that time is to get permission. Saying the relevant prayers in the morning is a tradition from Panchen Losang Chökyi Gyältsän; it is a method for somebody who forgets to seek permission at the actual time of the action to somehow receive fewer vices. In this way, one gets permission in the morning to do actions during the day such as sing or touch and keep things in one's house, to keep more food than is needed that day, to make fire and cook, to eat foods which have been gathered, etc. I am not sure that if one has done the prayers in the morning then at the time of actually doing these things it is all right to have worldly concern and not think it is for the sake of other sentient beings, for Dharma reasons. I think that to remember at the actual time is the main thing: that is why it is called "du ten" – remembering at the time. So, when a monk lights incense he should remember the gelong vow immediately - and think that it is for the sake of sentient beings, for Dharma practice. Then one will not degenerate the vows or receive vices.

When you light incense or a butter-lamp or some light, just before you offer it recite OM AH HUM each time, then offer it. There are various interferers, three hundred and sixty or something different dö-ens, who take the essence. Maybe that is, sort-of, their enjoyment. If one offers without blessing, one does receive the merit, but there is some interference in regard to the offering – it affects the mind, making it kind-of unclear or unstable. In order for these things to not happen one recites the mantra OM AH HUM and blesses the offerings.

You should cover your mouth in order to not pollute the offerings with smelly breath. His Holiness Serkong Rinpoche said the scarf should be white. We see the servants of the high lamas such as His Holiness the Dalai Lama cover their mouths with a white cloth or scarf when serving tea and so on. Also, the offerings are carried high. So when you make offerings in front of an altar you should not think, "I am just putting water in front of clay statues or pictures." You should act as if you are in front of a king or high lama and serving him. Due to our karmic obscurations we do not see the images as real, but Heruka is there, Tara is there, all the buddhas are there. The whole merit field is there, but due to karmic obscurations we do not see them. The karma that one has at the moment is to see merely pictures and statues of the deities. This is explained in the Lam-rim teachings, as well as by Pabongkha Dechen Nyingpo, I think, and His Holiness Trijang Rinpoche, His Holiness Ling Rinpoche, as well as Serkong Rinpoche.

The bowls should be placed neither touching nor too far apart. If they are too far apart, then due to that inauspiciousness or dependent arising one will be distant from the virtuous teacher in the future. So do not place them far apart, but also not touching. I think due to the dependent arising from placing them too close one will have a dull mind, without sharp intelligence. You should place them the distance of one rice grain apart. In regard to pouring the water His Holiness Song Rinpoche used to advise to first pour slowly, then faster, and then again slowly. Doing it that way does not make a loud splashing noise. If one puts too much water into the bowl and it overflows, one will have intelligence, but it will not be stable. One will easily forget or will not have a clear mind – things will get mixed up. One will not remember words or the meanings of things, or the meaning will get mixed up. Also, it may affect one's moral conduct so that it degenerates. Some bowls made in Nepal have lines to indicate how much water to offer in the bowl. About one grain-size of space should be left at the top, rather than filling it completely. That also makes it easier to not make a mess when you remove the bowls from the altar.

You can recite the mantra OM AH HUM again while you are offering, or the long mantra for blessing and multiplying the offerings:

OM NAMO BHAGAVATE VAJRA SARA PRAMARDANE /
TATHAGATAYA / ARHATE SAMYAKSAM BUDDHAYA /
TADYATHA / OM VAJRE VAJRE / MAHA VAJRE / MAHA
TEJA VAJRE / MAHA VIDYA VAJRE / MAHA BODHICHITTA
VAJRE / MAHA BODHI MÄNDO PASAM KRAMANA VAJRE /
SARVA KARMA AVARANA VISHO DHANA VAJRE SVAHA
(3x)

The benefit of reciting this is that not only are the offerings blessed, but clouds of offerings are received in front of each of the beings in the merit field. You can think in this way even at the very beginning of the offering. Whether you have Chakrasamvara, or Guru Shakyamuni, or Vajrasattva, or whatever, as your field of merit, think that what they see is nectar. To you it is water, but what the buddhas see is nectar. For a preta it is blood and pus, for us it is water; even the devas see it as nectar, so without question it is nectar for the buddhas who have completed the merit of transcendental wisdom and method. Think, "I'm offering them the nectar which appears to them."

While you are offering, think that whatever pictures or statues of guru-deities you have are the embodiment of all buddhas of the ten directions, the embodiment of the guru, of all three refuges, and that you are offering to all of them and that it generates infinite bliss in their minds. As explained above, offer the water bowls to every single holy object and actual living buddha and bodhisattva in the ten directions. You can concentrate on this while you are offering. As you are filling the bowls, with your mouth recite the mantra for blessing, with your mind offer to all of them.

After you have finished a set of offerings you can do the same meditation of offering over again.

His Holiness Serkong Tsenshab Rinpoche used to advise that at the end you should dedicate the merit in this way,"May this merit from making offerings..." – and all the merit accumulated by me and all other sentient beings – "not be experienced by me but rather only by other sentient beings."

Rinpoche's specific advice is to pray that the merit and whatever resultant happiness will come from that be received and experienced by other sentient beings, and that oneself not experience it. You should think like that. Each time, dedicate for the generation of bodhichitta with the prayer "Jang chhub sem chhog rinpoche..." even if you do other dedications; then it becomes a practice of the five powers of thought training. Accumulating merit in order to generate bodhichitta is the practice of the power of the white seed. You should dedicate the merit to achieve enlightenment quickly and more quickly for the sake of all sentient beings in whatever way you know.

Guidelines for Completing 100,000 Water Bowl Offerings

[The practice of offering 100,000 water bowls is one of nine preliminary practices or "ngöndros" performed in the Tibetan Buddhist tradition. The preliminary practices are designed to accumulate merit
and purify negativities in order to quickly generate realizations on the
path. They are also done in preparation for longer tantric retreats.
The nine preliminaries are to do 100,000 repetitions related to the
following practices: prostrations, mandala offerings, guru yoga, Vajrasattva, Damtsig Dorje, Dorje Khadro, tsa-tsas, water bowl offerings,
and refuge.]

When you do a hundred thousand water bowl offerings offer them
inside if it is easier. If not, then at the beach! Fill the whole beach with
bowls! Then, maybe the next day you will be taken to an institution
or a psychologist! If it is difficult to bring water repeatedly from some
distance then go to a place having water such as a river and set up the
bowls on a big board. That may be easier. When it rains it may be even
easier as you will not have to pour water! You just put the bowls out!
When you clean the bowls each day you should clean them well, not
just patting them with the towel. You must clean them well, not leav-
ing them damp. Not doing it just like giving them a sort-of blessing! If
there are any stains you should try to clean them with sand or other
cleaning materials.

   You can begin with the refuge and bodhichitta prayer "Sang gyä
chhö dang…" Then, on the basis of the Lama Chöpa or the elaborate

Ganden Lha Gyäma,* [do the practice from the beginning up until the limb of offering during the seven-limb practice]; then, make the offerings by setting out fifty, or one hundred or more, bowls at the offering section of the seven-limb practice. [Do the meditation for offering using the Extensive Offering Practice found in this booklet on pages 22–26], then make a dedication. Then, you pour out the water and rinse the bowls with water. Begin again with "Sang gyä chhö dang..." and then just do the offering section of the seven-limb practice, [fill up the bowls,] and again do the meditation of offering. Again make the dedication, and then pour out the water. Then perform the offering again, etc.

[Performing the offerings in a way that is,] "Beautifully performed, without being crooked," could mean performing the external offerings in a symmetrical way; but the main thing is to do it without having a crooked mind, which means making the offerings without being stained by worldly concern.

[When you have finished offering however many rounds of water bowls you are going to offer, then complete the remaining limbs of the seven-limb prayer together with the other prayers and meditations left in your practice text (Lama Chöpa or Ganden Lha Gyäma). It is very good to accompany your preliminary practice with meditation on the lam-rim. This can be done at the time of reciting either the "Lam-Rim Prayer" or the "Foundation of All Good Qualities" found in the Lama Chöpa and Ganden Lha Gyäma, respectively. It is also recommended at the end of each day of practice to do extensive dedication prayers as found in Essential Buddhist Prayers, An FPMT Prayer Book, Vol. 1.]

Lama Chöpa and Ganden Lha Gyäma (Lama Tsongkhapa Guru Yoga) practices can be obtained from the Foundation Store, www.fpmt.org/shop.

Extensive Offering Practice

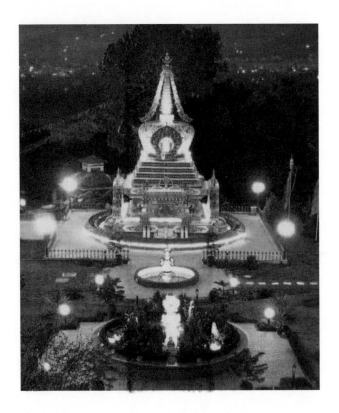

To Accumulate the Most Extensive Merit

composed by Lama Zopa Rinpoche

Extensive Offering Practice

A practice to accumulate the most extensive merit with lights and other offerings

Composed by Lama Zopa Rinpoche

Motivation

Before beginning your extensive offering practice, generate bodhichitta in the following way (if you are specifically doing a light offering practice, then also recite the words in parantheses):

The purpose of my life is not only to solve my own problems and gain happiness for myself but to free all beings from their problems and lead them to all happiness, especially the state of full enlightenment. Therefore, I myself must first achieve complete enlightenment. To do this, I must complete the two accumulations – the merit of fortune [method] and the merit of wisdom. Therefore, I am going to make charity of these (light) offerings and make offerings (of these lights) to the merit field.

Also remember to motivate for the success of particular projects, for people who have passed away or are sick, or for other specific purposes. Then generate the mind of refuge and bodhichitta.

Blessing the Offerings

Bless your offerings by reciting OM AH HUM three times. If you are making light offerings in particular, now light the candles or switch on the electricity while reciting:

OM AH HUM (3x)

In general, if you don't bless offerings immediately, they can be entered by the possessing spirit Tse-bu chig-pa, and then making those offerings can create obstacles for you; it can cause mental damage. In the case of possessed light offerings, without control, you fall asleep when listening, reflecting, and meditating on the holy Dharma. Similarly, if you don't bless all other kinds of offering, various possessing spirits can enter them. Making those offerings can then damage your mind and create obstacles for you.

Making Charity to the Beings of the Six Realms

Think that you have received these offerings through the kindness of all sentient beings. Think, "These offerings are not mine." Make charity of the offerings to all the hell beings, pretas, animals, humans, asuras, and suras. This is done to counteract the thought that the offerings belong to you. Think that you are making these offerings on their behalf – you and all other beings are going to make offerings to the buddhas together. Generate great happiness at having accumulated infinite merit by thinking in this way.

Also, think that these offerings are given to every sentient being of each of the six realms, becoming whatever they need for both temporary and ultimate happiness.

Offering to the Merit Field

I actually make and mentally transform the offerings of humans and devas. May Samantabhadra clouds of offerings pervade the whole sky.

Offering Cloud Mantra
This mantra multiplies the offerings so that they become numberless.

OM NAMO BHAGAVATE VAJRA SARA PRAMARDANE /
TATHAGATAYA / ARHATE SAMYAKSAM BUDDHAYA /
TADYATHA / OM VAJRE VAJRE / MAHA VAJRE / MAHA
TEJA VAJRE / MAHA VIDYA VAJRE / MAHA BODHICHITTA
VAJRE / MAHA BODHI MÄNDO PASAM KRAMANA VAJRE /
SARVA KARMA AVARANA VISHO DHANA VAJRE SVAHA
(3x)

Extensive Power of Truth

By the power of truth of the Three Rare Sublime Ones,
The blessings of all the buddhas and bodhisattvas,
The great wealth of the completed two collections, and the sphere of
  phenomena being pure and inconceivable;
May these piles of clouds of offerings arising through transformation
  by the bodhisattvas Arya Samantabhadra, Manjushri, and so forth
  – unimaginable and inexhaustible, equaling the sky – arise and, in
  the eyes of the buddhas and bodhisattvas of the ten directions, be
  received.

Presenting the Offerings

Make offerings to all holy objects, visualizing them as manifestations of your own root Guru, who is one with all other virtuous friends. Since the virtuous friend is the most powerful object in the merit field, by offering like this, you accumulate the most extensive merit. In his text, The Five Stages, the Savior Nagarjuna said, "Abandon making other offerings; try purely to make offerings only to your Guru. By pleasing your Guru, you will achieve the sublime wisdom of the omniscient mind."

In the root tantric text Buddhaya, Guru Vajradhara said, "The merit accumulated by making offerings to just one pore of the spiritual master is more sublime than all that accumulated by making offerings to all the buddhas and bodhisattvas of the ten directions." As you make the offerings, think that you are prostrating, making offerings, and that the Guru's holy mind experiences great bliss.

Place your hands in prostration mudra at your heart. Each time you make offerings, think that, "Having received the offering, the Guru's holy mind experiences great bliss." This completes the offering.

First, we make offerings to all the holy objects here in this place, every single thangka, statue, stupa, scripture, picture, tsa-tsa, relic, and prayer wheel, by seeing them as inseparable from our own virtuous friend, who is one with all other virtuous friends. (*Prostrate, offer, and generate great bliss.*)

Then, we make all these offerings both real and visualized to every single holy object in this country – all the statues, stupas, scriptures, pictures, all the centers' altars, every single altar in peoples' homes, the prayer wheels, tsa-tsas, and any virtuous friend in this country, by seeing them as inseparable from one's own virtuous friend. We present these offerings many times and in this way generate great bliss in all the holy minds. *(Prostrate, offer, and generate great bliss.)*

Then, we make all these offerings, both real and visualized, to every single holy object in India, including the Bodhgaya stupa where 1000 buddhas descended. Also we make offerings to all the holy beings in India, including His Holiness the Dalai Lama and other virtuous friends that you have there. By seeing them as inseparable from one's own virtuous friend, we make the offerings many times and in this way generate great bliss in all the holy minds. *(Prostrate, offer, and generate great bliss.)*

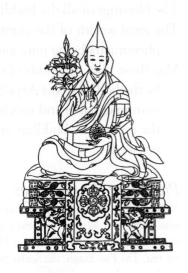

We make all these offerings, both real and visualized, to every single holy object in Tibet, including the Jowo Rinpoche in Lhasa that was blessed by Guru Shakyamuni Buddha himself, by seeing them as inseparable from one's own virtuous friend. We make the offerings many times and in this way generate great bliss in all the holy minds. *(Prostrate, offer, and generate great bliss.)*

We make all these offerings, both real and visualized, to every single holy object in Nepal, including Bouddhanath Stupa and Swayambhunath Stupa and any virtuous friends in Nepal. By seeing them as inseparable from one's own virtuous friend, we make the offerings many times and in this way generate great bliss in all the holy minds. *(Prostrate, offer, and generate great bliss.)*

We make all these offerings, both real and visualized, to every single holy object in the other Buddhist countries such as mainland China, Thailand, Taiwan, Burma, etc., by seeing all the holy objects as inseparable from one's own virtuous friend. We make the offerings many times and in this way generate great bliss in all the holy minds. *(Prostrate, offer, and generate great bliss.)*

We now make all these offerings, both real and visualized, to every single holy object in the rest of the world, by seeing all the holy objects as inseparable from one's own virtuous friend. We make the offerings many times and in this way generate great bliss in all the holy minds. *(Prostrate, offer, and generate great bliss.)*

We make all these offerings both real and visualized to all the ten direction Buddha, Dharma, and Sangha by seeing all of them as inseparable from one's own virtuous friend. We make the offerings many times and in this way generate great bliss in all the holy minds. *(Prostrate, offer, and generate great bliss.)*

We make all these offerings, both real and visualized, to all the ten direction statues, stupas, and scriptures by seeing them as inseparable from one's own virtuous friend. Make the offerings many times and in this way generate great bliss in all the holy minds. *(Prostrate, offer, and generate great bliss.)*

We make all these offerings, both real and visualized, to Buddha Chenrezig, by seeing Chenrezig as inseparable from His Holiness the Dalai Lama and one's own virtuous friend. Make the offerings many times and in this way generate great bliss in all the holy minds. *(Prostrate, offer, and generate great bliss.)*

We make all these offerings, both real and visualized, to the seven Medicine Buddhas (which is the same as making offerings to all the buddhas) by seeing them as inseparable from one's own virtuous friend. We make the offerings many times and in this way generate great bliss in all the holy minds. *(Prostrate, offer, and generate great bliss.)*

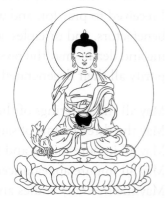

Then, we make all these offerings, both real and visualized, to the bodhisattva Kshitigarbha by seeing him as inseparable from one's own

virtuous friend. Make the offerings many times and in this way generate great bliss in all the holy minds. *(Prostrate, offer, and generate great bliss.)*

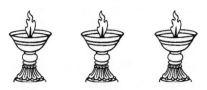

The Actual (Light) Offering Prayer

Now recite the actual prayer of the (light) offerings – five, ten, one thousand times, or however many times possible – depending on how many times you want to make the offerings:

These actually performed and mentally imagined (light) offerings, the
manifestations of one's own innate awareness, the dharmakaya, these
clouds of offerings equaling the infinite sky, I am offering to all the
gurus and the Three Rare Sublime Ones, and to all the statues, stupas,
and scriptures, all of which are manifestations of the Guru.

I have accumulated infinite merit by having generated bodhichitta,
having made charity to the sentient beings, and having made the actual (light) offerings to the gurus, Triple Gem, and to all holy objects
of the ten directions.

Due to this merit, whomever I promised to pray for, whose name
I received to pray for, and whoever prays to me – principally servants,
benefactors, and disciples, as well as all remaining sentient beings, living and dead – may the rays of the light of the five wisdoms completely
purify all their degenerated vows and samaya right now.

May all the sufferings of the evil-gone realms cease right now.
May the three realms of samsara be emptied right now.
May all impure minds and their obscurations be purified.
May all impure appearances be purified.
May the five holy bodies and wisdom spontaneously arise.

At this point, one may also recite Atisha's Light Offering Prayer as many times as one wishes *(see p. 60).*

Dedication

Ge wa di yi nyur du dag
Due to the merits of these virtuous actions
La ma sang gyä drub gyur nä
May I quickly attain the state of a Guru-Buddha
Dro wa chig kyang ma lü pa
And lead all living beings, without exception
De yi sa la gö par shog
Into that enlightened state.

Jang chhub sem chhog rin po chhe
May the supreme jewel bodhichitta
Ma kyi pa nam kye gyur chig
That has not arisen, arise and grow;
Kye pa nam pa me pa yang
And may that which has arisen not diminish,
Gong nä gong du phel war shog
But increase more and more.

Due to these infinite merits, may whatever sufferings sentient beings have ripen on me right now. May whatever happiness and virtue I have accumulated, including all the realizations of the path and the highest goal enlightenment, be received by each hell being, preta, animal, human, asura, and sura right now.

Having dedicated in this way, you have accumulated infinite merit, so rejoice.

May the precious sublime thought of enlightenment, the source of all success and happiness for myself and all other sentient beings, be generated without even a second's delay. May that which has been generated increase more and more without degeneration.

Due to all the merits of the three times collected by me, buddhas, bodhisattvas and all other sentient beings, which are empty from their own side, may the I, which is empty from its own side, achieve enlightenment, which is empty from its own side, and lead all sentient beings, who are empty from their own side, to that enlightenment, by myself alone.

Whatever white virtues I have thus created, I dedicate as causes enabling me to uphold the holy Dharma of scriptures and insights and to fulfill without exception all the prayers and deeds of all the buddhas and bodhisattvas of the three times.

By the force of this merit, in all my lives may I never be parted from Mahayana's four spheres, and may I reach the end of my journey along the paths of renunciation, bodhichitta, the pure view, and the two stages.

Light Offering Prayer

Composed by Lama Atisha

One may recite this prayer when making an individual light offering, or in the context of the Extensive Offering Practice. After lighting a candle, a butter lamp, or any form of light, this prayer can be recited in conjunction with the visualization described below.

May the light of the lamp be equal to the great three thousand worlds and their environments.
May the wick of the lamp be equal to the king of mountains – Mount Meru.
May the butter be equal to the infinite ocean.
May there be billions of trillions of lamps in the presence of each and every buddha.

May the light illuminate the darkness of ignorance of all sentient beings
From the peak of samsara down to the most torturous hell,
Whereby they can see directly and clearly all the ten directions'
Buddhas and bodhisattvas and their pure lands.

OM VAJRA ALOKE AH HUM

E MA HO

I offer these beautifully exalted clear and luminous lights
To the thousand buddhas of the fortunate eon,
To all the buddhas and bodhisattvas of the infinite pure lands and of the ten directions,

To all the gurus, meditation deities, dakas, dakinis, dharma protec-
tors, and the assembly of deities of all mandalas.

Due to this, may my father, mother, and all sentient beings in this life
and in all their future lives,
Be able to see directly the actual pure lands of the complete and per-
fect buddhas,
May they unify with Buddha Amitabha in inseparable oneness,
Please bless me and may my prayers be actualized as soon as possible,
Due to the power of the truth of the Triple Gem and the assembly of
deities of the three roots.

TADYATHA OM PÄNCHA GRIYA AVA BODHANI SVAHA (7x)

Visualization

The light transforms into single brilliant five-color wisdom.
On a lotus and moon disk the syllables OM and DHI appear.
From them, one hundred and eight beautiful goddesses of light,
Marmema, appear, wearing beautiful garments and precious gar-
lands.
Every goddess holds lights in her hands and from them emanate bil-
lions of trillions of infinite replicas of light-offering goddesses.
All of them make light offerings uninterruptedly to all the buddhas in
the buddhafields throughout all of space and to the peaceful and
wrathful deities.

Dedication

Thus, due to the merits of having made such a light offering
May all the benefactors, the deceased and migrating beings of the six
realms benefit;
May all their degenerated samaya and broken vows be restored;
May all their superstitious obscurations be purified;
May all their bad karma, negativities, and obscurations be purified;
May the three realms of samsara become empty immediately.
Please grant control, power, and realization.

Appendix
How to Fill a Small Statue

List of Materials
* Mantra strips for rolling (available from materials@fpmt.org)
* Stick incense to wrap the mantra sheets around
* Tape
* Yellow cloth to wrap around the mantra rolls and seal the statue
* Powdered incense to fill the statue
* If you have extra jewels or other precious objects you would like to offer to the statue, these may be included inside the statue too.

How to Fill the Statue
* Gently cover the face of the statue with cotton wool to protect it.
* Thoroughly wash the inside of the statue with mild dish soap.
* Cut out the mantra strips.
* Break a piece of incense to fit the short side of the mantra strip.
* Tightly roll one sheet of mantras onto the incense stick (note which way is up). Start with the head of the mantra sheet, not the end.
* When you have rolled 3/4s of the sheet onto the stick, place another sheet against the roll and continue rolling.
* Continue like this until your roll is the right size to fit snugly inside the bore of your statue.
* Tape the roll closed and mark which way is up.
* Wrap a strip of yellow cloth around the outside of the mantra roll and insert it right side up into the statue bore.
* Fill the base of the statue with powdered incense, jewels, etc. Fill the statue as tightly as possible so there is no empty space left.
* Tuck a piece of yellow cloth securely around the contents of the base, so they don't fall out when the statue is turned upright.
* Perform the short *Rab Nä* ritual (available from materials@fpmt.org) to bless your statue.

Colophons:

"Altar Set-up and Water Bowl Offerings" compiled by Ven. Gyalten Mindrol from advice given by Lama Zopa Rinpoche, and from Ven. Sarah Thresher and Kendall Magnussen in the FPMT Ritual Training.

"The Practice of Making Offerings" and "Guidelines for Completing 100,000 Water Bowl Offerings" were extracted from teachings given by Lama Zopa Rinpoche in a commentary to the Ganden Lha Gyäma given during the Second Enlightenment Experience Celebration in Dharamsala, India, March 1986. Provided courtesy of the Lama Yeshe Wisdom Archive (www.lamayeshe.com). Clarifying additions in "[ ]" and light editing by Kendall Magnussen, FPMT Education Department, May 2004.

"Extensive Offering Practice" originally composed by Lama Zopa Rinpoche in Taiwan in February 1994. Lightly edited for publication by Ven.erable Constance Miller and made available by FPMT Education Department, May 1998. That version was edited further and included as an appendix in Teachings from the Vajrasattva Retreat, Lama Yeshe Wisdom Archive, 2000. Revised edition, August 2001. Further revisions made by Kendall Magnussen, FPMT Education Department, April 2003 and Ven. Gyalten Mindrol, 2006.

"Light Offering Prayer" was composed by Lama Atisha and translated by Venerable Pemba Sherpa.

"How to Fill a Small Statue" compiled by Ven. Gyalten Mindrol, based on advice from Lama Zopa Rinpoche.

Foundation for the Preservation of the Mahayana Tradition

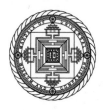

The Foundation for the Preservation of the Mahayana Tradition (FPMT) is a dynamic worldwide organization devoted to education and public service. Established by Lama Thubten Yeshe and Lama Zopa Rinpoche, FPMT touches the lives of beings all over the world. In the early 1970s, young Westerners inspired by the intelligence and practicality of the Buddhist approach made contact with these lamas in Nepal and the organization was born. Now encompassing over 150 Dharma centers, projects, social services and publishing houses in thirty-three countries, we continue to bring the enlightened message of compassion, wisdom, and peace to the world.

We invite you to join us in our work to develop compassion around the world! Visit our website at www.fpmt.org to find a center near you, a study program suited to your needs, practice materials, meditation supplies, sacred art, and online teachings. We offer a membership program with benefits such as Mandala magazine and discounts at the online Foundation Store. And check out some of the vast projects Lama Zopa Rinpoche has developed to preserve the Mahayana tradition and help end suffering in the world today. Lastly, never hesitate to contact us if we can be of service to you.

Foundation for the Preservation of the Mahayana Tradition
1632 SE 11th Avenue
Portland, OR 97214 USA
(503) 808-1588

www.fpmt.org

Foundation for the Preservation of the Mahayana Tradition